I0438813

KISS THE REFLECTION

Ideas, insights & imaginings on sending our
love cascading across time & space.

KISS THE REFLECTION

Ideas, insights & imaginings on sending our love cascading across time & space.

by

Daniel Sky Feather

ISBN 1-58500-897-4

1stbooks - rev.02/09/00

ABOUT THE BOOK

Who is this book for? It's for anyone who has ever ached for someone they love, anyone who has ever lost a loved one, either through death or separation of any kind. *It is for the soul who simply cannot stop loving, despite the absence of the one they love.* The most enduring pain the human heart could ever endure, is a feeling that love is trapped and without means of expression. This book offers unique and creative ways to continue expressing and transmitting that love when all other means of communication are no longer available.

Do you feel lost and cut-off from someone you love more than life itself? Do you dream about that special someone you have yet to meet? Are you grieving the death or loss of someone you love? Do you wish to send love back through time and heal your precious inner child? Are you in a relationship, yet feel more alone than you ever felt in your life? Are you in a relationship, and want to find ways to increase the magic you already feel for your lover? Or, are you simply looking for unique insights into setting the magic, the beauty, and the love in you, totally free?

If you answered "yes" to any of the above questions, then you are invited to walk with the author through the pages of this book. Maybe you will discover your truest love? Maybe you will discover the wings to your heart? Maybe your perspective, your very life, will never be the same again?

To my brother Tony,

whose love in my life is incredibly real.

"And any instant it wants, it can remember who it is, it can remember reality, it can remember Love.   In that instant, everything changes..."

Richard Bach
A Bridge Across Forever, a love story.
pp. 357-58

TABLE OF CONTENTS

PERSONAL IDEAS & INSIGHTS ON SETTING MY HEART COMPLETELY FREE 121

AFTERTHOUGHTS 129

INTRODUCTION

Whether the space that love must cross is between lips, or between vast distances, it still must travel through the mysterious gap which seems to set us apart from each other. And consider time, in relation to a kiss. The impulse to kiss erupts in each heart and mind, and the two lovers join their lips in a sweet exchange of energy. Yet, split seconds of time are standing between them: their brains must receive the sensations from their bodies, and then process the feeling back throughout their bodies. So, it seems love must leap over these split seconds, or dance over lifetimes, years, or even centuries, to make the journey from one heart, to the next.

This book is about expressing our love, communicating our love, and setting our love completely free, even where other forms of communication are not available. When there are no fax machines, email addresses, telephones, satellite transmissions, or P.O. boxes to send our love to, our hearts still long to continue loving. When there is no opportunity to speak, to touch, to hug, to make love, our hearts still long to continue loving. When our loved ones are ripped from our lives through tragedy and death, our hearts scream in agony to continue loving. *There is no way our hearts could ever stop loving, and the feeling that love is trapped or without expression causes the deepest pain human beings ever must endure.*

I will use the word "seems" many times throughout this book, mainly to illustrate a point, a subtle shift, in your internal reference that time and space, you and me, here and there, when and where, all just *seem* to be significant to the grand scheme of things. Just because we may seem alone, doesn't necessarily mean we are alone. Just because someone we love seems far away, doesn't necessarily mean they are. Just because it seems that grief and sadness will never cease, doesn't mean the pain will never end. What seems to be real, may not be real at all. *So, look beneath what seems to be real, and allow yourself the magical discovery of something more profound, more potent, more intensely joyous, ecstatic, and blissful.*   The true joy of living exists beneath what may seem real in the moment.

Lester Levenson, creator of the famed "Sedona Method®" for releasing and letting-go of limited feelings and beliefs, said once, "*Look for the perfection where the seeming imperfection seems to be.*" I invite you to do the same as you read this book. Look for the magic and freedom of your love where the seeming separation seems to be, or better yet, let-go and allow the magic and freedom of your love to blossom where the seeming separation seems to be.

In this spirit, I give great applause and thanks to everyone at Sedona Training Associates® in Sedona Arizona, for their excellence in teaching others the simple beauty of letting-go. The simple techniques I learned from their tape course, literally transformed my writing, and set this book free to create itself.

The path leading up to the creation of this book, for me, has been a diverse and eclectic one.

From the days in early February, 1987, when I walked back through the doors of recovery after going on my last drunk with tears brimming in my eyes and a five day beard, to the blissful joy of week long intensive workshops of personal healing, community building, ecology, and spirituality, my path has been filled with the deepest pain, and the most heightened ecstasy.

From the time the sun came over the mountains of southern Colorado to warm my drunken tears of self-pity, to the grueling 12-hour days of my 1st year in law school, I have always wondered and delved deeply into the meaning of life. Why am I here? What is going on? What is causing me to be here and breathing this moment? I have always been a curious seeker, and as far as my journey has taken me, I know this: *I don't know exactly how I came to be here, but I know that love is why I'm here. To love! To leap over mountains and dance with the moment, to love!* And I know I don't have to fully understand life, to bathe deeply in the bliss of this moment.

From the time I was 12 years old when my father grasped my brother "Peebs" and me in his arms and dropped the cruel news that our beautiful brother and hero, Tony, was killed in a motorcycle accident, to the time I stood bathed in the midnight sun of Alaska and wrote a poem to someone I loved, I have always known that my journey, my brief dance upon this earth, is to love. In the caverns of my deepest pain, to the exhilaration of that Alaskan sunset that wouldn't end, I have always sought to discover the magic of love. It's like a gold mine that never runs dry as long as I give it all away! *And it's also an energy, a sweet intoxicating energy that buzzes and hums, tickles and tingles throughout my mind and body as it is communicated, expressed, and transmitted.*

The spirit of my brother, his piercing beautiful eyes and golden curls of hair, shines luminously inside my mind, my memories, and my soul. And, I believe, his spirit also shines through the pages of this book. He taught me more, *beyond his death,* through his gentle, subtle nudging and the love he has so freely given me, (*which now, as I write, cascades freely down my spinal column to every cell in my body, causing tears of joy and love to fall upon the pages of my soul*) than he did in the short sixteen years he danced upon this earth.

From the time I stopped at every church I saw in England and Scotland to pray upon my knees, to my more evolved self dancing wildly and playfully to the beat of a drum around a sacred fire, singing ancient songs of healing and renewal, love has always been the thread which I have woven through all my experiences. *Love is all that matters.* It bridges culture, religion, time, space, yesterday, here, now, and tomorrow. My "church" is now my breath, the trees, the dance of the stream, the seductive movement of earth and star and moon, and the Mystery woven into it all. And my "religion" is love, itself.

When I sit next to a stream, the water doesn't ask me what religion I belong to. The water simply flows, and its sounds nourish and nurture my heart and mind, wiping away any remaining confusion about why I am here: *to simply love.* In this spirit, I offer these pages as a reflection of my own heart, to the world.

Maybe somewhere along the pages that follow, you too, will remember love, will remember who you are?

As you take each step along the path of your own bliss, as you are carried upon the notes of your own song, may you live, may you dream, and work, and play. . .

And may you take long deep baths in the bliss of the moment.

IDEAS ON HOW TO USE THIS BOOK

absorb the energy

Just as you read the words, paragraphs, and pages that follow, allow yourself to *also* absorb the energy as well. I wrote each piece with my left, non-dominant hand, which, I believe, creates a flow of energy from a deeper place in my heart, than if I were to write with my right hand. It is the energy, the love within me, that I extend to you. The words are merely the vessel.

So, I invite you to open your heart, take several pauses throughout this book, imagine love escaping your heart and soul, and notice the subtle changes in your awareness. Remember, just as a butterfly may, with her magical wings, alter the flow of wind, so can a small, subtle shift in your heart's awareness change the course of your life, forever.

reach over death

If someone you love has passed beyond death, and you are suffering from a grief and pain that feels like it will never end, then these ideas and insights will give you ways to continue expressing and transmitting the love in you that aches for freedom. You can miss them, and you can grieve, but you no longer have to suffer from the pain of feeling your love is trapped without expression.

As you read and absorb this book, just imagine that they are reading it with you, as they are within the same mirror reflection of love, that you are. As you feel and express your love for them in the coming pages, then they, wherever the feet of their soul may be carrying them, will also be reflecting back to you the beauty that is their love for you.

touch your soul-mate

Does your heart ache for someone you have yet to meet? Do you feel totally and madly in love with a dream of someone? Do you just know that your hearts must cross paths soon? If you are a romantic dreamer, and continue to allow your heart to dream despite the practical advice of others, then maybe you will meet face to face, heart to heart, breath to breath, soul to soul, with your cosmic lover as you walk with me along this rich, beautiful path of imagination?

Gently bring the image, or the feeling, of your future lover into that sacred space your heart knows all to well, and allow the magic of your love to naturally well up from the depths of your heart. She, or he, will feel you, and your hearts will be drawn to each other like giant magnets. *There will be nothing to keep you from meeting, if you totally believe in the power of love.*

a past relationship

Do you feel you have already met your soul-mate, and now, through whatever circumstance, you are apart again, with no idea how you will ever meet again? Do you feel like you have "blown it" and ache for a clean slate, for one more chance? Do you hope and dream she or he will forgive you and accept you into their heart again? If so, then send love to that place beyond time, beyond anger and conflict, beyond personalities, beyond hang-ups and emotional baggage, and then let-go and see what happens.

It may be best to simply let each other go, with love, and know that *as we let go, we are trusting that we are naturally woven into the greater magic of love.*

inner child

Are you recovering from a trauma so unspeakable from your childhood, that the stored pain is sabotaging your chance at true happiness as an adult? Are you in therapy recovering from childhood abuse of any kind? If so, these ideas and insights can be an invaluable tool for riding the magic carpet of your imagination back through the years to rescue your child, and ultimately free yourself.

You can hold and love the child, in you, that has nobody else to turn to, who is hidden in the darkest closet of time. You can bring this precious, magical, broken child into this moment, where you are right now, where it is safe, where there is light and happiness and healing.

your ideal future self

If you are constantly dreaming and working toward a future where you are financially, physically, mentally, emotionally, and totally free in every respect, then take pen to paper and create your perfect future. Let the image of what you may look like and where you might live, i.e., a beautiful house, totally healthy, color and radiance in your face, etc. Then, use these ideas and insights to send love to your future self! This energy, this love, will form a connection between the two of you, and your life will begin to naturally merge together as one.

In this way you are building a bridge, closing the gap, and making your path of *becoming* joyous, effortless, and real.

enemy

Pick out the person in your life that you literally "hate" to deal with, or that it seems you hate, or who irritates you, or who grates on your nerves like fingernails on a chalkboard! Secretly use this person as the one you love across time & space. The sweetest "revenge" you can offer up an "enemy" is to let go of the identification of yourself _as_ their enemy, and quietly convert yourself, within your heart and mind, into their friend.

You will be amazed at how this simple shift in your internal reference can totally transform their behavior and attitudes. Or, maybe they won't change at all! At least you have let them go, and set your heart free to focus on other things, rather than on how much they irritate you.

lovers

Okay, so you're already immersed in a blissful union with someone you love. If each of you undertake to journey through this book individually, following along and imagining love cascading to each other, then your joy may just rupture into ecstasy!

alone in a relationship

Are you in a relationship that is leaving you feeling *more alone*, than if you were totally by yourself? The measure of intimacy is not determined by physical closeness alone, but rather by the openness, the vulnerability, and the freedom by which the energy of your love flows. It's truly baffling to be in a relationship and feel more alone than you ever felt in your life.

If this is the case, then these ideas and insights may in fact be the catalyst for re-lighting the spark of passion in your relationship. Use this book, secretly, to shift your internal perspective about yourself and your mate, and then let-go and see what happens.

love transmissions and magical questions

In each section, there will be *love transmissions* and *magical questions* for you to contemplate upon. In each case, simply allow them to be reflected into the mirror of your own soul. Experience them from the place in your heart that doesn't make sense.

Take several deep breaths, and release the tension in your body. Allow your heart and your mind to settle. Gently focus your mind and allow your awareness to relax, and feel your heart begin to open and expand. The effect of doing this, is a feeling of experiencing life from a subtle sense of being larger than life.

When thought and love are combined in such magical ways, the result is a flow of timeless, beautiful energy. So allow the love transmissions to be messages of love you extend, and the magical questions to be energy you release within yourself.

In truth, your heart, and the timeless magic it contains, *really is larger than life.* So don't just read this book, delve into it, experience it. By doing this, you are delving into yourself, into your own sense of magic, into your own sense of Beingness, and into your own dance with the Divine.

When you set the love transmissions and magical questions free, they are released into your subconscious mind, and into a deeper place in you. They will then reflect back to you the pure magic contained in the Mystery of your soul.

any other way

Use this book in any other way to dissolve the seeming sense of separation between your heart, and the hearts of others, the heart of the Universe itself. *Could it be that you have never,*

ever, been separated, and your real journey is about remembering love, remembering yourself, remembering your freedom?

remember this

As we journey together through the pages of this book, remember this: *love transforms the lover, as the lover transmits love.* So in all the moments of your life, be a lover, make the conscious choice to remember your love, to remember the beauty and freedom of your heart, and what before was a sense of "far away" will happily and effortlessly dissolve into joy.

AWAKENING & REMEMBERING THE TIMELESS FREEDOM OF OUR LOVE

What difference does distance make?

Scientists and mystics are discovering something truly remarkable and spectacular about the concept of distance. They are finding out that, although there seems to be vast space and great distance between particles on each "side" of the Universe, distance is not relevant to the particles themselves. Each particle seems to be intrinsically aware of what the other is up to. So, the question, then, is this: *What difference does it make how "far apart" they might be?*

Maybe it doesn't matter at all?

Let's carry this strange truth into matters of the heart, into the idea of sending love to someone who feels, to you, that they are far away. *First,* thought, by its very nature, is intuitively and intrinsically aware of thought, regardless of "where" or "when" thought occurs. *Second,* what has kept us from realizing and remembering the brilliant power of our thoughts, is fear. We have been taught to be afraid of ourselves, of our brilliance, our beauty, our natural authentic power.

Yet, what is easy to grasp onto, is also easy to let go of. Just as naturally as we fear ourselves, we can let go of fearing ourselves.

Can you imagine the boundaries which would dissolve if all of us, all at once, remembered the beauty and power of our thoughts?

Love transmissions

What is easy to grasp onto, is also easy to let go of. It is a simple and easy decision to let go of being afraid my own greatness: the power of my mind, combined with the power of my love.

Magical Questions

*Am I willing to let go
of being afraid of my own brilliant intelligence?*

*Am I willing to remember how strong and beautiful
my love really is?*

Sacred imagination

Walk with me through this imaginary dance:

Thoughts of love are simply not subject to the illusionary laws of time & space. *Thus*. . . My own loving thoughts are free to travel to any place and any time in this beautifully orchestrated universe. *Thus*. . . I find that space, time, tomorrow, yesterday, here, and there are but crafty *constructs* of my thoughts. *And*. . . My mind encompasses the universe. An exploration of the whole universe is but a magical journey inside the movement of thought. *And*. . . Love is the purpose of my thoughts, of my Beingness. Therefore. . . *Love is any "where" and any "time" I choose to imagine love to be.*

Love transmissions

Love is where or when my beautiful, rich, fluid mind imagines love to be.

Magical Questions

Where or when would I lovingly choose to imagine love to be?

Tears into water

Consider for a moment, how water is connected. It doesn't cling, or grasp, or hold on, or attempt to control. It continually lets go, and in this fluid act of surrender, it is connected to everything.

Water transmits the bliss of love to the human heart. In any given moment, water may be apart from water. Yet, it is never separate. The water in your body, or the water in a glass, has in its cells a patient awareness that it will *always* return to a state of blissful, fluid union. *The tears you shed will eventually find their way back to the depth of the ocean.*

Go to the nearest stream, or body of water. Sit and listen for awhile. Let your thoughts naturally find the person you love. Let your love for them build in your heart, and, if you so choose, let your love overflow as tears.

As you think of them, and feel the enormous beauty of your love for them, let the water of your tears fall and magically blend into the waters' stillness, or the waters' movement, and say, "*I love you. These words I speak, are beyond space, beyond time.*" Keep repeating these words as you continue blending your tears with the sacred waters of the Earth.

Then trust that the sacred waters will carry the beauty of your tears, to their heart.

Love transmissions

As my tears, my love, my sorrow, the precious innocence of my heart, mixes and blends with the waters of the earth, the music that is my love will echo and cascade throughout your being.

Magical Questions

*Does the act of placing my tears into the waters of the earth
set my love free?*

Moon remembers

Throughout the unfolding of human history, can you imagine how much love the moon has witnessed? The magic of the first embrace, the sweet love making, the aching sorrow of separation, all happened under the loving, watchful eyes of the moon. If the moon has witnessed love unfold across the ages of human history, then the moon can transmit our love across those ages. *The moon offers you a most beautiful way to send love.*

During the next full moon, go out upon the soft green earth. Stand, and gaze into the face of the moon. Relax, and breathe deeply.

Let your heart fill.

Let your heart overflow. Open the palms of your hand to the light of the moon, and speak your love. Let the words of your heart flow luminously from your lips! If you feel the palms of your hands getting warm, then you know your love is being transmitted to one you love.

Wherever they are along their journey, the same moon you are speaking your love to, is cascading the magic of your love upon their heart & soul.

Can you see the soft glow of moonlight upon their face? Warming their heart and soul?

Love transmissions

As I send my sweetest love to the full, pregnant moon, I choose to believe the moon will nurture your most precious dreams.

Magical Questions

If I spoke my love to the fullness of the moon, could I choose to believe that my love will be conveyed across time & space?

Your own eyes

We each exist within the hearts of each other, like circles within circles, stretching into tomorrow and yesterday, here and there, all within the dance life's sweet, captivating moment. We can get so "caught up" on sending love to those "out there" that we seem to forget that everyone we love finds their real existence within our own heart and soul.

Find a mirror. Light two candles, and place one on each side of the mirror. Hold your hands softly over your heart and gaze deeply into your own eyes.

Imagine the person you love, is you, and you, are the person you love. Speak these words to the one you love as you peer into your own eyes:

The person I love is me, and I am the person I love.

Keep repeating this circular affirmation as you gaze into your own eyes. Look deep into their/your eyes. Express your love to them/you as many times as your heart wishes to speak the words.

This meditative exercise can be enormously intense and powerful, so be prepared for a possible deep, cathartic emotional release.

Love transmissions

The shortest path to loving you, is to bathe myself in the precious love I wish to extend. We exist in each other's heart, so you will experience the love I shower upon myself. To love you, I choose to love myself.

Magical Questions

Am I willing to bathe myself in the love I hold
for _____?

Is the greatest gift I bestow upon others the full and
unconditional love I give myself?

Do my loved ones want me, more than anything, to truly love
myself?

Kisses in the wind

On a windy day, go outside and kiss the palm of your own hand. Kiss your hand as softly, and as sweetly, as you would the person you love.

Blow the kiss into the wind and say, *"Behold, my love for thee, is free."* Imagine your kisses are carried onto the winds that encircle the Earth. . . Into the winds of light and energy that traverse millions of miles in seconds. Kisses, carried by the winds of air and time and energy, will playfully dance like butterflies along the sweet, fertile landscape of eternity.

Keep blowing your kisses into the wind. Keep reciting the sacred words of your love for as long as your heart so desires.

Love transmissions

*As I blow my kisses unto the sweet winds of forever, the love
I feel will freely dance above time, to caress your heart with joy.*

Magical Questions

Could I blow my kisses across time, across distance, as easily and as
playfully as I could, across the room?

Let go

Sometimes, it can be hard to let go. When your body, mind, and soul <u>wants</u> them <u>so</u> <u>bad</u>, the ache and the wanting *itself* can make you feel more isolated and disconnected from them.

Imagine this. . . You are standing on the edge of a great cliff. The waves of an endless ocean crash into the rocks below. You hold your love in your hand.

Do you see your hand? Is it closed tight, holding onto them with all your heart's might? If you are, *it's okay*. It's natural to hold on, but remember, it's also a natural human ability to release, to let go with trust and love.

In one act of love, in one act of trust, of freedom, open your hand. Open your mind. Open your heart. Open your soul, and let your love for them be free. Let your love for them go. It doesn't mean you stop loving them. In fact, love is stronger, when love is set free. It's a paradox, that when embraced, produces a feeling of intimacy with life, just as it *also* sets you free to love on deeper and deeper levels.

Can you see the butterflies of all shapes and sizes and colors escaping the palm of your hand and launching out over the sea? Can you see these butterflies finding your loved one with playful ease and joy? Can you see these butterflies tickling them with the tiny winds from their tiny wings?

Love transmissions

I choose to be courageous, and let go. I choose to trust, and let go. The love I set free, will circle through eternity and back, to find my heart that set love free.

Magical Questions

Does my longing for someone, my wanting him or her so bad, seem to push him or her away? Could I choose to simply let them go?

If this frightens me, could I embrace my fear with love? What if true togetherness is a never-ending willingness to let each other go?

Music of silence

Interwoven among the many millions of sounds all around us, is a Silence with a music all its own. Connecting to this Silence can be simple and effortless.

Practice listening in a *whole way* to all the sounds around you, at once. Absorb all the sounds with an open mind, and you will tune in to the musical Silence that is the heartbeat of everything.

Listening to the sounds of Nature, of birds and animals, and the wind through the leaves of the trees, is *especially effective* in tuning your inner mind to the Silence.

While embraced in this sacred silence, think of the one you love. Let your love, and your heart, and your mind, and your body, dissolve completely into Quiet.

Then, imagine the same Quiet dissolving into them.

Love transmissions

Silence transmits the magic of my love to forever and back again, like the Womb of Life embracing all life in peace, in joy, in rest, in remembrance, in new magical beginnings.

Silence is the music of love.

Magical Questions

What messages of love does Silence convey to my open heart?

Could I offer the whole of my love back to this Silence?

The palm of your hands

In a physical sense, the way we touch another, is with our hands. In a deeper sense, our hands convey our love, and communicate our tenderness. How many of us have wished for just one more touch, one more hug, one more kiss, with someone we seem to have lost? *Of all the things about them, it's their touch we miss the most.*

Our hands can send the energy of our love out over the span of distance, and touch the hearts of those we love.

To do this, bring to your mind and to your heart, the image of someone you love, physically present in your life or not, that you ache for, and feel apart from. On a separate page an image of them in the center, or write a poem to them and place it there, or simply write their name.

Once this is done, place your hands gently upon the page, barely touching it. Imagine your hands are feathers, resting softly upon their soul. Then let go, and allow the precious love in your heart to fill, and to overflow. *Give yourself to the love, to this moment, here and now.* Allow yourself total freedom to cry, to grieve, to shed your tears, to laugh, or to sing.

Let your hands rest upon the page and send them love for as long as your heart so desires.

Love transmissions

As my hands convey love across all distance, I can allow my emotions to simply be, to have wings and nourish, cleanse, and wipe away the silly illusion that love, mine and yours, could ever be separated.

Magical Questions

Could I let go, totally and completely, and allow my hands to convey my love across time & space?

Tears within tears, within tears

What *are* tears, but raindrops falling from the sky of our souls, from the dance of the Mystery, from the sweet laughter of Eternity?   We spend too much time hiding our tears and disguising our pain, that we forget to celebrate the beauty of those tears.

I once road my bike down the road, crying and sobbing with complete abandon.   People looked at me strangely.   Yet, the wind on my face seemed to celebrate my tears as it gently cooled my face.   As terrible as I felt at the time, I felt a strange freedom encompassing me.

If you give yourself to your tears, and allow your tears the freedom to fly, they will shed their skin and reveal even deeper tears.   Whether they are tears of love, of celebration, joy, grief, anguish, or aching sorrow, they contain a deeper magic, a mirror, a window across time and distance, death and loss, and seeming separation.

If you choose, and if your heart is so ready and open, allow your tears to shed, to fall from your eyes.   Place the sweet moisture upon your fingers and drop them onto, and into, the space that seems to exist between your heart, and theirs.   Let your lips utter the words "I love you," and your love will fall like raindrops from the sky of their own precious dreams.   A tingle of joy will magically erupt inside their being.

Love transmissions

The tears I offer you, in freedom to the sky, will carry my love over and beyond what I once thought was far away.

Magical Questions

Could I trust the freedom within my tears?

Get up and dance

At a week-long healing retreat deep in the Mark Twain National Forest, I was curled into a fetal position, pouring the unspeakable pain of loss into the soft, moist soil beneath me. As I thought about my brother Tony who died when I was young, my body shivered and sweat poured off my forehead. I was touching and embracing the core of my sorrow.

Everyone else was getting up, moving about, beginning to dance, and singing a strange, hypnotically happy song of celebration. I didn't want to get up. I wanted to stay within my pain. *There was comfort and safety in the depth of my sorrow.*

Yet, with the help of others, I curled out of my fetal position, stood, and with the words choking through my pain, I joined in the song and began to dance. My feet stepped with a renewed energy, and a renewed joy. It was as if the celebration of life was *breathing a cool refreshing wind through the caverns of my deepest grief and sorrow.* My brother, whom was ripped from my heart so many years earlier, seemed to be dancing with me, within me, in that beautiful moment.

Can you allow yourself the courage to touch and embrace the core of your sorrow? Can you go one step further and allow yourself the courage, after you have shed your tears, to get up and dance?

Love transmissions

The moment that follows my deepest sorrow, in which I choose to dance, will breathe through me and awaken in me the sweet freedom of my love.

Magical Questions

Is their sorrow in me I have yet to embrace?

Could I then get up and dance in sweet celebration
for the miracle of this living moment?

Whisper

Whispers carry love across time & space.

The next time you are in bed, and just as your drift into sleep, whisper your love into the night. Make it a seductive whisper that penetrates dreams, that easily floats onto the wind and instantly finds the ears of your lover.

Continue to whisper your love to them as you fall asleep. Your whispers will lull you into a magical, fantastic night of dreams.

Whisper the words, *I love you_____, I love you_____ I love you_____.*

Repeat this until your whispering within the fluid movement of your dreams and each word of love you speak gives birth to starlight and stardust that magically causes whatever feelings of separation to vanish, instantly.

Love transmissions

As I whisper words of love into my dreams, my dreams will carry those sweet whispers effortlessly into your soul. Whispers are the magic carpet of my love.

Magical Questions

What few words of love would my heart choose to whisper
to someone I love who seems far away?

Love's reflection

What if you, upon the moment of your death, found yourself at a door? When you walk in, you find yourself in a strange kind of observatory. Instead of looking up, you are looking back down into a reflection of a still body of water. You see your funeral. Everybody is crying, and grieving your loss.

"I wonder what that's all about," you may ask yourself. All of it, every single piece of life's drama, exists within this reflection, where from this vantage point, you see, has no separation.

You also know it is completely okay for your loved ones to be crying. Grief is a process for the soul's awakening to love. They would not be grieving unless something inside them knew, that you are still with them, and will be joined with them again along the path of eternity.

Inside the core of sorrow, are the seeds of knowing that love, will find love, once again. And deep inside the core of grief, are tears of utter and complete joy.

Maybe you will cry, too? Maybe yours will be tears of joy because you are looking back upon the reflection of life, knowing there is no separation.

Imagine your tears falling into the still pond, sending ripples of pure love across the surface of the reflection. Inside each beautiful soul you loved during your brief dance on earth, a tingling ripple of joy will cascade throughout their being.

Love transmissions

If I take an imaginary journey beyond the moment of my own death. . . then look back, I will see no separation in the reflection of my love.

Magical Questions

One moment beyond my death, what words would I speak directly into the hearts of those I love?

Surrender the illusion of control

You are bound to this moment of life that sets your soul ablaze, and the wings of your heart to the freedom of the wind. In any given moment, are you willing to surrender your illusion of controlling your surroundings, other people, and situations?

Within your willingness to surrender control, if only for a timeless instant, is also the willingness to allow joy and ecstasy to catch you, to embrace you, to reveal your unlimited capacity to remember the true freedom of love.

Maybe magic, and joy, and love, can just happen? Effortlessly?

It's a strange sort of paradox, that when embraced, fills the soul with joy: *In surrendering the illusion of control, all the love you once tried to force with all your might, will magically and abundantly flow in colors more brilliant than you previously imagined.* It's called the magic of surrender, of letting go, to let love and beauty become you.

Don't try to force love through time & space. Instead, surrender to life this moment, and allow with an open, effortless, joyous heart, the greatness of love to simply *be*, in you.

It's so easy to want to become someone. But wouldn't you need to be first, before you become? What about just stopping along the path of your journey and allowing love and joy and a sense of utter connection to find and embrace you?

Love transmissions

I allow myself to release the illusion that the beauty of love's flow could ever be controlled. I breathe, relax, and rest into this moment right now, and allow love to simply be.

Magical Questions

Could I let go of trying to control the beauty and freedom of love's flow?

Sacred Breathing

The simple act of breathing is your connection, your intimacy, your life. You can go weeks without food, and days without water. However, you can only go minutes without air.

Your breath is the energy of love.

Think, for a moment, very closely to the following question.

How could I ever feel alone, when every breath I exhale, is inhaled by a beautiful tree, and every breath exhaled by a tree, is inhaled by me?

The same is true for souls who love each other across time and space. They inhale every breath of love you exhale, and you are continually breathing in their love for you, whether you are conscious of it or not. It's all a great, rhythmic, fluid exchange.

Look into the eyes of this fluid, breathing moment of your life. Surrender to its beauty. Savor its mystery, its joy, and its love. Can you embrace the freedom it offers you?

Love transmissions

What I exchange with the Whole, I exchange with you, whom I love across time & space. My every breath is a symbol of this beautiful exchange.

Magical Questions

*Could I breathe with the awareness that my love is being
exchanged freely with the whole of life?*

Big

I once had a dream that I was placed in a type of machine that put me into an immediate, deep sleep. I woke surrounded by stars: so bright, so intense and so close, that I could reach out and touch them. Someone else was there: *someone I loved.* We joined hands and danced among the stars, tears falling from our souls, to form more stars, and more stars, and more, and more. . .

Think yourself big. Imagine your body is as large as galaxies. You can fly through space with the power of your love. Is there any place, with your love, you cannot go? Is there any place, or any time, outside the reach of your love?

Love transmissions

I allow my awareness to expand clear to the touch of starlight where a single droplet of my love gallops and sings through the galaxies with ease and laughter and joy.

Magical Questions

Could I think? Then observe myself thinking?
Then witness myself, observing myself thinking?
Could I expand my awareness and encompass the earth, the sun
the stars, even the galaxies in the precious greatness of my love?

River of Tears

Imagine for a moment, that your tears fall from your soul, to form a river of loving energy *just* beneath the level of consciousness.

Can you see this river flowing under the surface of conscious understanding?

Can you see this beauty that is your tears, pushing upward through the soil of the heart and soul of the one you love?

Can you see springs of pure love welling from within their mind, from within their thoughts?

Can you see flowers of ecstasy bursting and blossoming inside them?

Can you see birds and butterflies dancing about?

Let go, and allow yourself to see, or to feel, your tears nourishing the seeds of their joy.

Love transmissions

I allow my tears to fall from my soul and nourish the seeds of joy and beauty in your heart, "where" ever or "when" ever you might be.

Magical Questions

*Could I allow the precious, timeless energy of my tears
to nourish the beauty in another?*

Free

Do you feel distant from your soul-mate? Maybe you already met, and now have parted ways again? Maybe you are yet to meet? Is it frustrating to not know when you will meet again?

Your soul-mate wants you to love freely. It is okay to be apart from your soul-mate for many, many lifetimes, because the love you share, enfolds all lifetimes! Every person you love, *your soul-mate shares in that love.* That is the freedom in love. You can let your soul-mate go, and let her go a million times, because somewhere in you is the knowledge that you will always be together, regardless of how "far" you may be from her.

Maybe time "apart" is the best time soul-mates ever spend together? Love freely, and love with abandon.

Love transmissions

I don't wish to <u>save</u> my love for some far away time. I choose to <u>share</u> my love with life, now. I choose to pour my love into the moment, to dance wildly with life.

You may seem far away, yet, you wish for me to love freely, because you will share that love, as you are forever within each living breath of my soul.

Magical Questions

Could I celebrate the love I share with my soul-mate
by letting go?
Could I then choose to pour my love into the
sacred cup of this moment?

A perfect moment in time

Take a deep, full breath, and allow everything that you see going on around you, and everything you feel spinning within you, to slow down. . . into a perfect. . . moment. . . in time.

Ordinary moments can be perfect too. If you are sitting in a bookstore drinking coffee, watching everyone around you talk among themselves, slow it all down and allow this moment to become full and blossoming and perfect. If you are reading a book on a Sunday afternoon, taking a walk through a big city, or by a lake, or simply thinking of someone you love, allow your awareness to slow down, and for this moment to blend into shear, complete perfection.

Everything, this moment, is as it should be. Love is the breath, that connects us all. We are in rhythm with the heartbeat of the earth, the stars, and the moon. We are not looking in upon nature and admiring Her beauty. *We are nature.* We are the breath, the beauty, the droplet of rain, and the drifting clouds. Every element that makes up our body, makes up the stars, the soil, the wind, and the water.

We are the love that propels the magic of creation spiraling blissfully forward.

The simple truth that you are living is enough to allow this moment, this instant you are reading these words, to be complete, full, perfect, beautiful, and timeless.

Love transmissions

I now slow my thoughts down, seductively down into cool, gentle stillness. . . and immerse my mind and heart into this stillness. This moment is perfect, and stretches into forever, rippling love into your beautiful heart & soul.

Magical Questions

Could I allow my whole life to be one perfect, fluid moment?

Sit and wait

To connect your love to anyone, anywhere, sit and wait. Do nothing else. *What if the one you are loving across time & space, is also loving you?*

If this is the case, the surest way <u>for</u> <u>them</u> to feel your love is to open your heart, to <u>theirs</u>. It is a simple truth, and a simple paradox: *That which you seek, seek not and wait. That which you once sought, has always sought you, and now has the freedom to find you.*

Let's now translate that into the language of the heart: *The one you miss, misses you. If you stop searching for them, they will find you. Their love will find you. Once their love finds you, yours will enfold them.*

Love transmissions

I now open my heart to receive your love. . . knowing that <u>my love</u> will then happily embrace your soul.

Magical Questions

*Could I open my heart like a flower to the sun
and allow myself to receive the beautiful warmth
of the love I wish to give?*

More than goodbye, more than hello

Are you beginning to feel excited and ecstatic at the thought that *time and space, although seeming to exist, holds no significance to the human heart that embraces the freedom of its love?*

That time and space are merely toys for the playful soul to further awaken love's awakening, like a song blossoming as a flower?

Maybe our souls choose to live in bodies and die and be born, love and lose, meet and part, in order to further this blossom?

Think about this. . . *What about actually celebrating the distance that seems to exist between your souls?* Maybe this is a way to dispel the illusion of being separated?

Agonize the distance, and the distance seems to persist.

Celebrate the distance, and the significance of distance dissolves.

In the arms of goodbye is the next magical hello, just as in the arms of death is the seeds of re-birth. Distance is actually a dance between souls who know, at their core, they can never be separated.

Love transmissions

In love's awakening is my growing awareness that we, both of us, are more than goodbye, and more than hello. We are love's intelligence. We are more than anything we ever imagined before.

As I celebrate whatever distance which seems to exist between us, I discover how boundless and free our love really is.

Magical Questions

Could I celebrate and honor the distance that seems to exist between me and the one(s) I love?

Laughter's sake

Laugh for the sake of laughter. Laugh yourself to tears. Laugh yourself to sleep. Laugh yourself awake. Laugh yourself to a delirious, acute, absolute mad sense of ecstasy!

Who ever said you need a reason to laugh?

Laughter knows not a single boundary. It ripples across the magic of total possibility to giggle inside the hearts of everyone you love, have loved, or ever will love.

Love transmissions

Laughter is the universal energy that time & space cannot comprehend or contain. Each day, I make a point to laugh for laughter's sake, allowing the music of my soul to soar over time & distance like rainbows of stardust.

Magical Questions

Could I give my laughter wings?

*Could I make appointments with myself throughout the day
to simply laugh?*

Naked

Be naked in the presence of life's moment, in the presence of love.

Stand, in your mind's imagination, naked unto a night filled with a billion (or so) brilliant stars. Spread your legs, dig the roots of your love into the soil of your awareness, hold your arms <u>up</u>, and your hands <u>open</u> <u>wide</u> to the universe.

Light is patient. As the light from stars many millions of miles away finally reaches your naked body, mind, and soul, then so does the brilliant light of your soul travel back to dance with all you see above.

To be naked, vulnerable, and exposed to the brilliant expanse of starlight, is to allow the piercing brilliance of your heart to penetrate space, penetrate time, and set your entire being ablaze.

Love transmissions

The naked light of my soul bathes the heavens in beauty. . . The galaxies and stars take notice of me, see me, and stand in <u>awe</u> of my beautiful light that exists forever without limitation or boundary.

Magical Questions

Could I allow my defenses to shed and be more vulnerable
and naked in the eyes of love?
How else could my beauty ever be seen?

The tree's perspective

Rest on your back, under a tree. Stare up into the sky, through her stretching green leaves. This is the trees perspective on love, and life.

Observe the backdrop of the sky mixing with the color of the leaves. Lose your focus. Let your vision blend. Let all the colors blend.

Peel your heart and your body wide open and let go. Release and relax all the muscles in your body in one beautiful act of surrender: to life, to the leaves, to the beauty, to the tree as she patiently opens her body to the sky.

Let your body and heart patiently stretch to the sky, as does the branches and the leaves. Let the whole experience become you, and joy will overwhelm your senses.

Love transmissions

As I gaze into the sky through the eyes of a tree, I let go, and allow the love in me to stretch above time & distance to embrace your heart with peace, serenity, and joy.

Magical Questions

*Could I allow my heart to be as patient in its expression
as the tree is in her peaceful stretch to the sky?*

Witness the Silence

Often there is a silence between souls. A still quiet. A rest.
A pause.

This does not mean that love is gone, only that love is resting.

Look with eyes of patient, *non-judgmental acceptance* at the distance that seems to appear between you and those you love.
Look in on your life. Become the sacred, loving witness.

Simultaneously witness life, and experience life. This will deepen your experience of life.

Love transmissions

I offer my love to the distance, and to the time, and to the Silence, between our souls.

Magical Questions

Could I let go, <u>into</u> Silence?
And welcome the peaceful Quiet that may exist
between myself
and someone I love?

Simple love

Love is simple, so perhaps, the easiest way to send love showering across time & space is as follows:

1. *Hold your "far away" loved one in your thoughts.*
2. *While they occupy your mind, allow your heart to fill and overflow with love.*

This combines the power of mind, with the power of the heart, with the power of love. Thought is pure energy, and the heart contains love, which is timeless.

Therefore, when thought and love are combined, an energy is formed which transcends boundary, and language, and culture, and time, and death, and distance, and anything else that seems to separate your souls.

Love transmissions

I magically blend my thoughts with my love. This combined power transcends everything, and embraces you with the warmth of my love.

Magical Questions

*Could I simply think of someone I love and then
allow my heart to overflow?*

Empty

Become empty, in body and in mind, and in soul. The instant you become empty, you fill to overflowing. The filling, and the emptying, is the ebb and flow of love, of the universe itself.

To be completely empty, is to overflow with love. To overflow with love, empty your mind and body.

The next time you are in bed, and ready to fall asleep, completely and deliberately let go of all the muscles in your body at once. Imagine all the energy in your body completely draining. See how many seconds you can stay in this totally empty and relaxed state. (Practice this often)

When you are empty and relaxed, think of the one you love. The emptiness in your mind and body, combined with your relaxed attention upon your lover, will create a rebound effect that will transcend the "laws" of time and space.

Nature will instantly fill the "vacuum" with energy, with love. In this way, your love will launch like fountains of light over and above your conscious understanding.

Love transmissions

I surrender to life and empty all my thoughts and energy into this blissful moment. Love then overflows and travels anywhere your heart may be. Emptiness fills my soul with ecstasy, and sends my love giggling across forever.

Magical Questions

Could I practice a state of total, blissful emptiness?
Then allow Nature to overflow all my sensations with love?

Dream butterfly

A purple and orange butterfly lands on the windowsill of your dreams. You may wonder why such a beautiful creature has graced your sleep time.

Then you realize something truly spectacular about the dream butterfly. *It can reach into dreams and beyond. It can change the course of hurricanes. And yes, it can carry love from a human heart to any place and any time in this imaginable universe.* One single *love thought*, carried to the sky, and let go, can change the course of human life, instantly and forever.

Imagine a tiny, shimmering bubble of white energy (your love) forming and escaping your mind. It floats over and rests gently upon the back of the butterfly. *You watch it lift off.* You see it lift above your house, above the trees, above the clouds, above the earth, above the stars, above time, and thought, and here, and there, and yesterday, and tomorrow. The butterfly carries the love clear above everything, above all that exists, and all that ever will be.

Then, guess what happens? The butterfly lets your love go, and the white bubble begins to drift lazily back down, into time, into forever, into the past, into tomorrow, and into the stars and clouds and. . .

Where "ever" or when "ever" your soul-mate, lover, or loved one finds their moment of existence, this bubble, which is now millions of bubbles, of your love, will shower them with a joy that is <u>as</u> sweet <u>as</u> <u>it</u> <u>is</u> timeless.

Love transmissions

I drop my loving thoughts upon the dream butterfly. . . Love carried to the sky, above everything and let go, will multiply, and fall, and drift, back into forever.

Magical Questions

What thoughts of love would I offer to the dream butterfly?
Could I trust that she will find her way?
And canvass my love upon forever?

I misplaced time

One day, I was going about my day as usual, and something very peculiar happened. *I misplaced time.* I simply *forgot* where I put it.

All the clocks disappeared, and I wandered through my life, as if in a dream. I wondered what time it was? I wondered what date it was? Or what year it was? Or what century it was? Or millennium it was?

I would sleep, and my night would burn like the sun, and the moon and stars would shimmer during the day. When I was awake, I dreamt. When I slept, I did the dishes. Everything seemed backward, upside down, inside out. *I wondered if I was off my rocker completely. Had the batteries in my brain fizzled into nothing?*

Then, one day, after a million years that never happened, *and* that lasted forever, had passed, I saw a strange ball of sunlight on my kitchen table. I walked closer, and looked into the ball of energy. I touched it, and through my body surged a laughing, tickling kind of *ecstasy* I had never known before.

Upon closer inspection, I saw time racing along inside the ball of light. Dates and events, deaths and births, loves and losses, grieving and joy, the whole drama of time seemed to be all be happening *at once*. Then, it hit me like a million stars bursting into light all at once. . .

Love transmissions

All time happens in the flash of one grand, timeless moment. As I look into the eyes of now, time is forgotten, and I remember forever. In forever, all the love I ever wished to speak or express, finds its destination, even before I utter the words and before the tears fall from my soul. . .

Magical Questions

Could I purposely misplace time and remember forever?
Would I then remember love, remember myself?

Eyes of love

The eyes of the universe, are the eyes of love, connecting soul to soul, from past to present to future, from here to there to everywhere, as a beautiful silk thread weaving human hearts into the tapestry of forever.

If you go outside on a brilliant clear night, and you lay on a blanket and gaze up into forever, you are gazing into the soul of love, the eyes of forever, the joy of *now*. As you do, it is <u>as</u> <u>if</u> you are gazing into the hearts and minds and eyes and bodies of everyone you ever loved, regardless of where, or when, they might be.

Stare into the eyes of a billion stars bursting into forever, and whisper the most famous, most potent words of all time, "I love you," and every "one" every "where" any "time" whom you have loved, or will love, will feel the sweet, intoxicating whisper of your love blowing through their souls.

Love transmissions

I stare into the eyes of the stars and love all I see. . . Love then penetrates all I cannot see.

Magical Questions

Whose eyes do I wish to gaze into the next time I look with awe and wonder at the beauty of the stars?

Infinity

In the center of a circle 8, is the point of beginning, of ending, now and forever, in the pulsating, ecstatic breath of this moment.

Think sweet thoughts of the one you love who seems far away or who seems in an other time, and then bring to focus the circle 8 and look at the center point.

Then spin the symbol in your mind. Allow yourself to see an infinite number of circle 8's forming in a trace like pattern, off the center point.

This image creates a doorway, a pathway, which leads from forever into now, and from now into forever, which are, in essence, the same.

Love transmissions

As I spin the circle eight in my mind, I see Infinity beginning in the end, and ending where it begins, ultimately finding its breath, its meaning, in love . . .

Magical Questions

Is my love like a circle 8, spiraling into forever
and spinning back into now?

Circle of forever

Time and love are but a circle within a circle, with neither a beginning, nor an ending. You can sit in the middle of this miracle, in the center of forever, and send love like a million duplicate postcards, to everyone. *The circle is the oldest, most timeless symbol of forever.*

Imagine, in your mind's eye, that with your finger, you draw a circle of white, sparkling stardust around you, to form a perfect circle. When your circle is formed, trace the stardust to all that is above you, all that is within you, and all that is below you.

When you are finished, say this aloud: *Behold, I am in the center of forever, where I am free, where my love is free!*

Then just *be*. Breathe. Allow all your thoughts to flow in, and flow out of your mind like a river of energy. Judge nothing. Observe yourself, from outside yourself, sitting in the center of this moment, the center of now, the center of joy, of freedom, of love.

Nothing is impossible when the circle of eternity embraces you.

When you are ready, think about this special one you love, across the room or across death, or across lifetimes, or across forever itself. Let their eyes, their light, their energy, their smells, the feel of their touch, their memory, or the dream of them, come to your mind, and to your heart. See, or hear, or feel, or sense them in any way your heart does choose. When you are ready, speak these words to them . . .

Love transmissions

In the center of this circle of time and beauty, I love you. Along the circle of eternity, I do send the essence of my love to you.

As this circle is forever, you are forever, and I am forever. My love for you is forever. Because our love is forever, I can let you go, and feel you, in the sacred journey of your soul, circling back to me.

Magical Questions

What words of love would I speak into the circle of
of time, love, and forever?

Two streams

There is a timeless place where souls meet, where souls join. It's like two streams dancing down the face of life. Their waters mix, and their waters merge. There is magic in the timelessness of their union. The moments they share push through the soil of immortality to rise like flowers in the sunshine of eternity.

Yet, the two streams may one day flow apart. But are each ever the same again? Their individual flows are greater, and stronger, and filled with more passion and beauty, than before they were joined.

Even though the streams may travel apart, and alone for many miles, many lifetimes, many joys and many sorrows, the timeless beauty of their union will continually and forever nourish them. Although the streams may not be flowing together, *the streams are still together*, because there will always be their union, way up the stream of yesterday, that is, and will always be, forever joined.

Think about the love you shared with someone who is no longer physically by your side. Enlarge the picture. Bathe in its joy, its magic, and its timelessness.

Love transmissions

Love, once shared, will <u>always</u> be shared. The place where the streams of our souls were joined to form a river, will always nourish my heart with love, strengthen me, and free me. I will always bathe in the timeless freedom of our moments.

Magical Questions

Could I allow the sweet memories of love shared to fill this moment, here and now, with freedom and joy?
If I can feel the love, now, that I once shared, then, doesn't that mean my heart is without time?

A bridge

Relax, and completely let go of every ounce of tension in your mind and body.

Imagine a bridge forming in your imagination, and disappearing into the mists of time & space. Imagine yourself stepping onto the bridge, and with each step, another piece of the bridge is built.

Are you willing to step with your thoughts into the air, risking the fall, with trust that your love will form a bridge for your soul to stand upon? To waltz and dance across time and space upon? *Remember,* that which you imagine, becomes real, inside you. What is real inside you, is all that matters anyway. Everything else is merely and illusion.

If you keep walking on this bridge, you will see that it climbs higher and higher into forever. When it begins to crest, allow yourself to look down. Isn't the view incredible? Can you see your very small, very insignificant little tiny problems that used to bother you so much? Can you see the garden of time? Can you see the reflection of your love in the realm of everyday life?

You are standing upon a rainbow, and this bridge continues on to the lives and hearts of everyone you love. From this vantage point, from this perspective, this state of heart and mind, everyone you even think about, will feel your love already.

Love transmissions

My imagination is a bridge upon which my love stretches above everything, into forever, into the gold within your heart.

Magical Questions

Could my imagination carry my love across continents, across lifetimes, across here and there, and clear across forever and back?

The holy grail

Have you ever searched for the holy grail, the sacred cup, to drink of the sustaining waters of life's mystery, to fill your being with the ecstasy that both feeds you <u>and</u> frees you?

Legend has it that King Arthur sent his greatest knights out in search of it. The search, itself, bled their souls dry and drove them clear out of their minds.

What did the Merlin do? He did nothing. He waited. He simply sat in his tree because he knew a wise truth: *that which ye seek, seeks thee.* So he let go of all thought and all desire to find the holy grail. Then a very strange miracle occurred: *the holy grail found him, because it <u>was</u> him.*

The human heart <u>is</u> the sacred cup, the holy chalice, and the love contained therein, is the sacred well. Drink of its waters. Let the simple joy of your love for life spill over the cup and fall from your soul as tears.

Then perform the magic of the holy grail: <u>drop</u> <u>those</u> <u>tears</u> <u>back</u> <u>into</u> <u>your</u> <u>heart</u>. This will ring a chime in the hearts of everyone you ever loved, and time & distance will become musical instruments for your souls to sing to each other with.

Love transmissions

The sacred well of my heart continually and eternally seeks me. I choose to wait . . . and let myself be found. It is here, within myself, that I drink of ecstasy . . . that my soul may dance again.

Magical Questions

Could I rest, stop searching, and allow the holy grail of my body and the sacred well of my love, to overwhelm my senses with ecstasy?

Whole being smile

A genuine *whole being* smile can shift consciousness, wash toxic thought from the soul, clear energy, and open channels of communication through the veil of time & space.

Start by letting your heart form a smile on its inner face. Let this energy move up your throat and into the back of your neck. Let it spread into your mind, behind your eyes, until your face turns itself "on" like a light bulb.

Then, go a step further, and let all the cells in your whole body relax, respond to this energy, and join in the smile.

Think of the person you love, and bathe them in the light from your whole being smile. Your beauty will be like orange light bathing the green rolling hills of their heart and mind.

Love transmissions

I choose to smile with every cell in my body, and every ounce of my soul.

Magical Questions

Could I bathe in the energy of a smile which spreads to all parts of my body, mind, and soul?

Forgive yourself

Maybe when you parted with your loved one, harsh painful words were exchanged, and life never afforded you the opportunity to apologize, forgive, and say *I love you* one last time? Maybe you regret the things you said and the way you acted in light of the way you *really feel* about them?

Is your love trapped in time, behind painful words and hard feelings?

In the eyes of your mind, think of your loved one, open your hands in a giving gesture, and say, *I love myself, forgive myself, and set myself free.* Then let all the energy in your body release at once.

Repeat this as often as you need.

When you forgive yourself, and set yourself totally free, you automatically forgive everyone you love, because they find their real existence within your heart.

Love transmissions

I choose to let go, forgive myself, and set myself free. When I do this, I also set you free. We exist within each other, so to forgive myself, is to set you free. There will be no need to forgive each other, if we forgive ourselves completely.

Magical Questions

Could I bathe myself in total forgiveness to set those I love completely free?

Kiss the reflection

There is a time when the moon begins her climb into fullness, when the evenings are gentle and quiet, and the land is silent, peaceful, and still.

The sun descends and the light begins her seductive dance with the coming night, and the moon comes out over the trees and begins her journey over the land of our dreams. In this special moment in Nature, you will find a quiet, still body of water. In this water, you will see the moons reflection, and you will know you are looking into life's reflection, and into the reflection of love, itself.

Kiss the tips of your fingers, and gently place your love upon the reflection.

Love transmissions

As I place my kisses upon life's reflection, I allow my lips speak the beauty of my soul: "As I kiss the reflection of life, I kiss all of life. As I kiss the reflection of love, I kiss all whom I ever loved, or ever will love. There is no separation in love's reflection."

Magical Questions

What magic awaits me when I place the beauty of my tears
into the pure reflection of life and love?

Unbutton your body

Your soul lives within the garment of your mind, and your mind lives within the garment of your body. Just as you unbutton your clothes to reveal the naked purity of your body, so can you unbutton your body to reveal mind, to reveal soul, to outpour love across the vastness of life.

Start at your forehead, and move down your body, *unbuttoning your body in a sacred act of offering your love to life*. Your body is merely a sacred garment that your soul, in its infinite journey of unfolding the brilliance of its love, has chosen to wear. With your imagination, you can unbutton your body and allow the love within, to flow free: *to continually unfold in a sweet seductive act of surrender.*

Continue to unbutton your body, all the way down to the tips of your toes. Can you feel the sparkling truth of your soul's love beginning to pour forth? A white river, sparkling with gold and silver and dust from the stars, finds its way, over mountains, over time, and over lifetimes, to offer your love to everyone.

Can you see this love pouring from your soul and forming an endless well before them? The freedom, then, is in the offering of love.

Love transmissions

Love, I am, for you. As I offer my love to you, with freedom, across time & space, the very love I offer, sets free, my own heart that set love free.

Magical Questions

Could I set myself free by offering the love that I am, to others, to life, to this moment, here and now?

PERSONAL IDEAS & INSIGHTS ON SETTING MY HEART COMPLETELY FREE

LOVE NOTES

What are my own creative ideas & insights on how I could send my love across time & space and set my heart completely free?

LOVE NOTES

LOVE NOTES

LOVE NOTES

LOVE NOTES

AFTERTHOUGHTS

Writing this book has been a fascinating process. As I wrote, and re-wrote the passages, I began to get the sneaking suspicion that this book was creating me!

What we create, with love, most always ends up creating us in the process. My awareness is a little more open to the freedom within me, and I hope your heart is a bit more open as well.

Daniel Sky Feather

ABOUT THE AUTHOR

Daniel Sky Feather is a writer who lives in Southwest Missouri. His healing journey began in 1987 after a long battle as an adolescent with drugs and alcohol. Along his path, he has participated in several week-long intensive workshops in the Mark Twain National Forest, cut off from the stresses associated with every day life, where he delved deeply into the interrelationships of ecology, psychology, and spirituality. Out of these very intense and transformational experiences, came a heightened awareness of love, a clear insight into the boundless freedom of the human heart, and an understanding of how to live in utter bliss by bathing in the magic and beauty that each moment of life offers us. His writing is a product of his profound personal journeys within himself.